LOREEN WILFRED

THE HAIR BIBLE

The Ultimate Guide to Hair Care, Discover Everything
About How to Take Care of Your Hair, How to Prevent Hair Loss
and Great Hairstyles That Would Work Best For You

Descrierea CIP a Bibliotecii Naționale a României
LOREEN WILFRED
    THE HAIR BIBLE. The Ultimate Guide to Hair Care, Discover Everything About How to Take Care of Your Hair, How to Prevent Hair Loss and Great Hairstyles That Would Work Best For You / Loreen Wilfred – Bucharest: Editura My Ebook, 2021
    ISBN

LOREEN WILFRED

THE HAIR BIBLE

**The Ultimate Guide to Hair Care, Discover Everything
About How to Take Care of Your Hair, How to Prevent Hair Loss
and Great Hairstyles That Would Work Best For You**

My Ebook Publishing House
Bucharest, 2021

TABLE OF CONTENTS

INTRODUCTION 7

Chapter 1. *Hair Style Basics* 9

Chapter 2. *Examine Your Face Shape* 12

Chapter 3. *Best Styles For An Oval Face* 16

Chapter 4. *Best Styles For A Long Face* 19

Chapter 5. *Best Styles For A Square Face* 22

Chapter 6. *Best Styles For A Round Face* 25

Chapter 7. *Best Styles For A Heart Shaped Face* 29

Chapter 8. *Learn To Love Your Style* 32

Chapter 9. *Hair Loss Tips* 35

Wrapping Up 48

INTRODUCTION

As though we didn't get adequate age betrayal from our faces, necks and hands, now we have to fret about it from our hair. However with these tips, you're aging locks will go from a boring gray to a healthy (vernal) shine! Get all the info you need here.

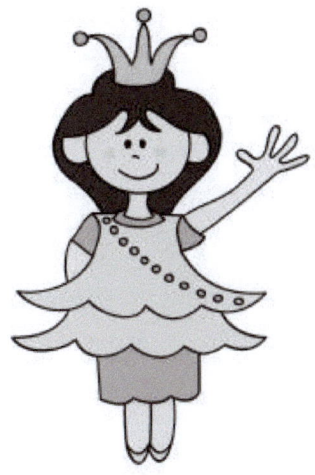

CHAPTER 1

HAIR STYLE BASICS

Synopsis

The basics for more youthful hair.

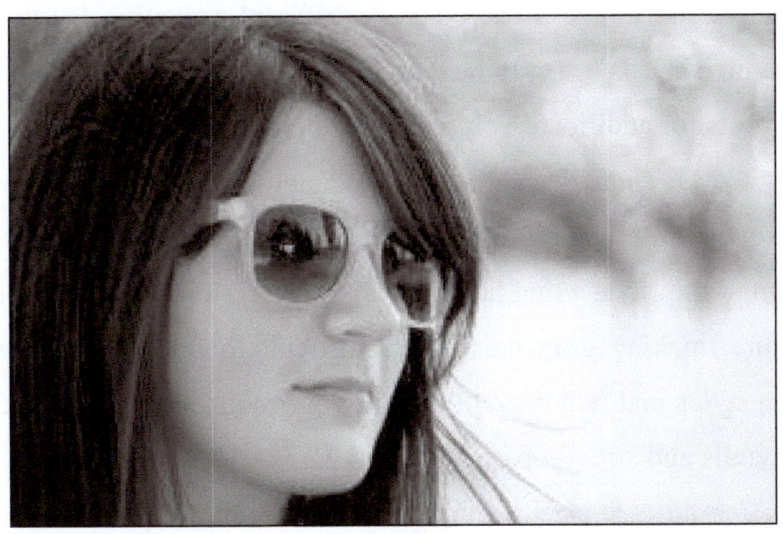

The Basics

Add Bulk – such as our male counterparts, we females have to fret about thinning hair also. If looking for styling products, seek supplements to fill out your strands. To beef up weakened hair, try taking a thousand micrograms of biotin and five hundred milligrams of niacin on a day-to-day basis. You might likewise wish to try a women's Rogaine solution twice a day to energize hair growth.

Volumize – utilize the oldest magic trick in the book if fighting thin, lax tresses: invest in an exceptional texturizing serum – and utilize it each day. A different exceptional way to volumize hair is to get to be a pro at teasing. Softly backcomb at the roots for additional volume at the top of your head.

Cover Those Dull Roots – Have age-promoting gray roots however can't make it to the beauty parlor till next week? For a prompt fix, style your hair in waves. Curls produce a deeper texture, making gray hairs more difficult to find. Keep away from styles that will brazenly flaunt your roots, like slicked back ponytails and straight parts.

Increase Shine – Shiny hair is exceedingly youthful and sexy. The simplest way to accomplish a boost of shine is through heated styling. All the same, make sure to apply a heat-protecting spray to your hair prior to utilizing, as you need to prevent harm to hair from heated styling equipment. If blow drying, utilize the concentrator attachment for greater aim directly down the shaft of your hair, assisting the cuticle to lay flat. Seal the cuticle with a flat iron or curling iron.

Shampoo Correctly – Washing hair may cause it to lose its glow after awhile. The medium shampoo and conditioner has a pH of 7, causing hair cuticles to pick up and fade in color. Utilize a shampoo with a pH approximately 4.5 and 6 to prevent this.

Preventative Steps – Everything we do to our hair (heat styling, dying/highlight, hair brushes, and so forth.) Finally do cause harm to its strength and durability. To fix as well as preclude this inevitable harm, attempt to wash your hair every other day instead of once a day, and air dry if possible.

Utilize anti-breakage, fortifying and restorative shampoos. These are more likely to see to it that ingredients produce layers on the hair shaft and seal split ends. Attempt to deep condition your hair on a weekly basis for a more saturated, hair smoothing experience.

CHAPTER 2

EXAMINE YOUR FACE SHAPE

Synopsis

Are you thinking of a new haircut or style? There are a lot of things you have to think about when selecting a fresh hair style, like: how much time you wish to spend maintaining a certain style, whether the texture of your hair will accommodate the hairstyle you've selected and lastly the shape of your face.

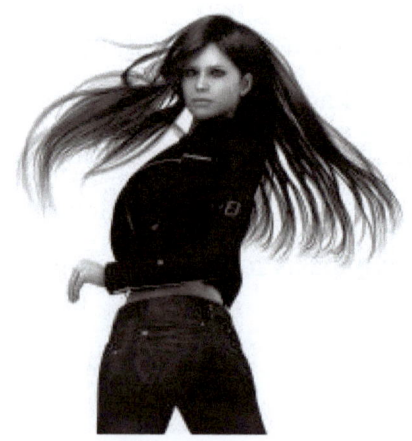

Face Shapes

This chapter will address picking out the correct style for your face shape.

The 1st thing to ascertain is the shape of your face and the simplest way to achieve this is:

Pull your hair back off your face and fasten it. Look directly into a mirror and outline your face with lipstick either right on the mirror or a sheet of transparent paper. A different choice is to take a photograph of you with your hair firmly tied back and outline the image.

Now examine the image closely and compare it to the assorted types of face shapes (circular, egg-shaped, square, triangle, oblong, heart, diamond). Although at first it could seem to match a couple of different shapes it's more than likely your face will be nearly resemble one shape over all others.

Circular Face - The round face has the same width brow as the lower face. Think about a circle which is the same width at the top as it is at the base. To boot round shaped faces have big cheeks.

You can stretch the face and minimize the fullness with a haircut that frames the face. As well as framing the face a side part or slender off center part helps downplay fullness. Long, streaming strands that cover the side of the face will temper the check bones and produce a longer well-defined illusion.

Square Face - The best length is 1 1/2 inches beneath the chin or shoulder length. In addition layered hair helps to cushion the jaw line. Think about parting your hair down one side with a side sweep to produce a different angle.

Face framing layers and a side part may likewise weaken an angular bone structure. Think about a shagged layered cut with a deep side part to counterbalance the strong angular characteristics.

Egg-shaped Face - think about an egg-shaped, the top and bottom are the same sizing with longer sides. Egg-shaped shaped faces may wear any style; all the same I advise that you have your hair away from the face and not to have too broad bangs.

All the same, regardless the length of your cut, you'll look better with layers near your cheekbones, lips or chin, essentially whatever feature you wish to highlight. Prevent short layers that add height on top of your head. This will make your face look long.

Heart Face - even as the name implies the face is wide at the cheekbones and brow and narrow at the jaw line. A side part with bangs and chin length or longer with layers will stretch the face. By ending the hair at the chin it renders the illusion of an egg-shaped face rather than a pointy chin.

Diamond Face - are broadest at cheekbones, and have a narrow forehead and jaw line of roughly equal widths. Think about a hairdo that adds width at the chin area like chin length bob cuts or shoulder length wisplike kicked out looks.

Haircuts that are styled tucked away behind the ears likewise work well to flaunt your wonderful cheek bone structure work well too. Likewise, think about square across bangs to shorten longer faces and side parts.

Oblong Face - Have high brows and long chins. In order to minimize the length of the face prevent hairdos that add a lot of volume at the top. Bangs are likewise great to shorten a long face.

CHAPTER 3

BEST STYLES FOR AN OVAL FACE

Synopsis

If you have an egg-shaped face shape, stop for a minute and congratulate yourself. You've landed the most versatile face shape. You may wear virtually any hairdo. So what are the best hairdos for egg-shaped faces?

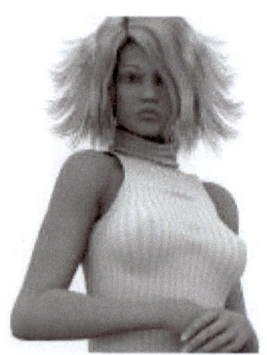

Oval

Regardless the length of your cut, you will look finest with layers close to your cheekbones, lips or chin; fundamentally whatever feature you wish to highlight.

Jennifer's Aniston's haircut looks amazing on an egg-shaped face. The long layers hit at the cheeks and the chin. The hair is longer in the back and shorter in the front so it does not weigh down Aniston's face. If you're petite, you need to prevent super long hair in the front as you run a risk looking like you're eleven years old.

As so many styles work for you, bear in mind these rules for coming up with the perfect hairdo for your personality and hair texture:

Rule 1: Stay away from dated hairdos. If you have not altered your style in 10 years, discover a fresh photo and get your hair cut. A foul hairdo may age you by many years (some celebrities prove my theory).

Rule 2: do not fight your natural hair texture. You may straighten out curly hair, but it takes time and cash. Why not invest in a great haircut for your curly hair as an alternative? If you have hyper- thin hair, do not try to grow your hair past your shoulders without the help of extensions, your hair will be dead and flat, regardless how much product you place in it. As an alternative, cut in layers and keep the length above your shoulders. Discover inspiration in shoulder-length hairdos.

Rule 3: If you're offbeat, get a funky hair cut and color. If you're a crazy busy mother, cut your hair so it's fashionable, yet does not require a quarter-hour a day of styling. Make certain your hairdo suits your personality and your life-style.

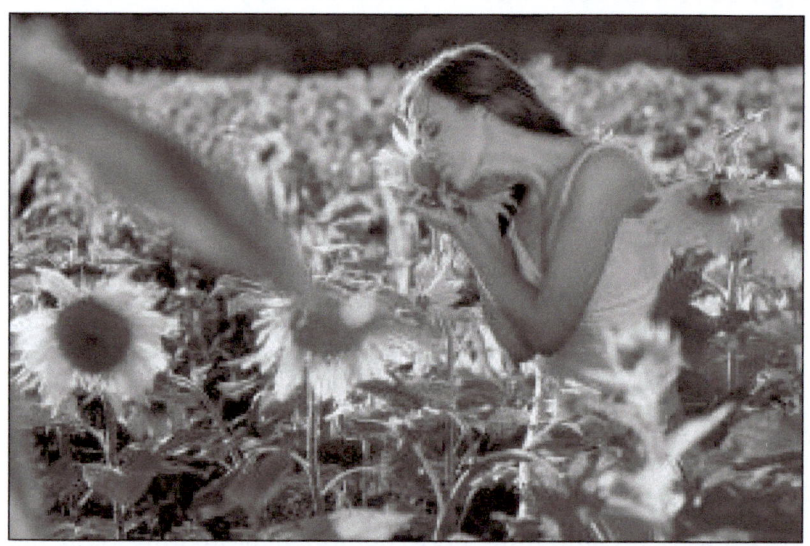

CHAPTER 4

BEST STYLES FOR A LONG FACE

Synopsis

If you, like me, have got a long face shape there are hairdos that look great and hairdos that look bad on you. Here are a few rules when thinking of a hairdo for a long (or "oblong" face shape):

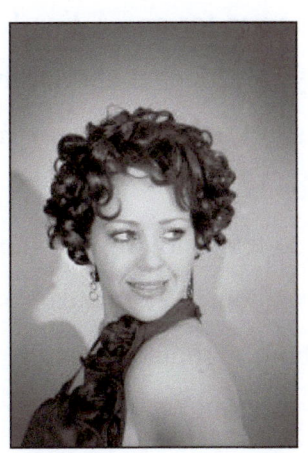

Long

1. If you have straight hair, you are able to produce more width with bangs. Bangs make your face seem shorter as they cover up an especially large forehead. You are able to wear anything from blunt bangs to longer, side-swept bangs.

2. Chin-length bobs and cuts are likewise ideal for you as they produce the deception of width.

3. Long, straight hair is commonly a no-no on a long face shape as it drags the face down. All the same, you are able to break this "no long hair" rule if you have waves or curls. Much body adds width to the sides of the face.

4. Think the uber-trendy long bob, which is really flattering on a long face. The length is important, and soft waves help. Ask your hairdresser for an "A-line Long Bob" where the back is approximately 1 1/2 inches shorter than the front.

5. If you love short hair, keep away from short layers that increase volume on top.

You don't want to let your hair grow too long if you have a long face shape. How come? It makes your long face appear super long. Think about a shoulder-length hairdo, like the one actress Asia Argento wears.

If you wish to have longer hair, cut it in long layers. The shortest layer ought to hit at your chin.

Short hair like a bob looks gorgeous on a long face. The bob ought to end at the jaw, chin or cheekbones to flaunt bone structure. The best bobs are shorter in the back and angle downward to the front. What I like about bobs are how modern and fresh they are.

Bangs work beautifully on a long face. There are examples of great bangs and bad bangs. Some bangs are too puffy and curled under. Some bangs are super cool and modernistic.

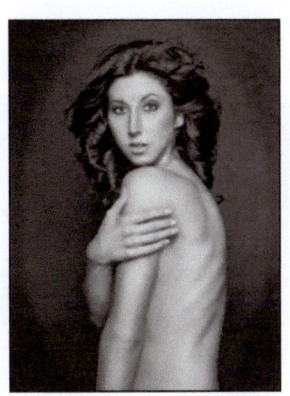

CHAPTER 5

BEST STYLES FOR A SQUARE FACE

Synopsis

If you have a square face you are likely wondering what style suits you best.

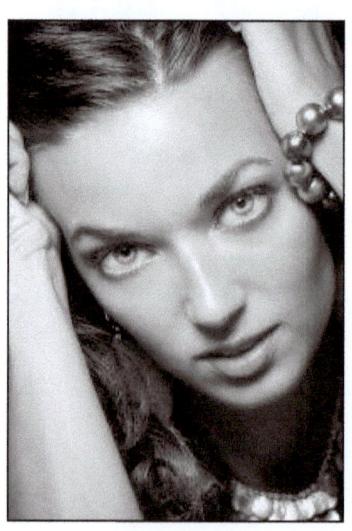

Square

Just following the birth of her son, Moses, Gwyneth Paltrow cut off her long hair which grew to her bosoms and plainly was too long (she acknowledged as much).

She tried a long bob for some time, however is now happy with a long cut that ceases below her collarbone. She parts her hair straight down the midsection, making what might be a boring look really modern. Make certain to cut in just a couple of long layers for motion.

Bobs are exceptional on a square face, as long as they're soft and layered. Keep away from a sharp, blunt bob, which will only accent your jaw, making the boxiness evident.

A wavelike style is perfect for a square face. The curls impart a softness, yet the short cut is still really edgy, much more so than the boring long locks.

In Good Housekeeping mag, New York styler Sean James Decuers states the pixie cut is most flattering on square faces (and ovals and hearts, as well).

Shoulder-length hairdos look exceptional on all face shapes. Rosario Dawson, a classic square face, wears a collarbone cut with waves. This look imparts softness to her strong jawline.

If you've any innate waves or curl to your hair, think about letting it go natural to cushion your angular features.

Jessica Simpson is a classic square face and her long hair is cut so bluntly on the base, you are able to see the straightness of the line. Long hair is really flattering on a square face; however make certain to ask your hairdresser to cut in a couple of long layers to add a little softness to the front.

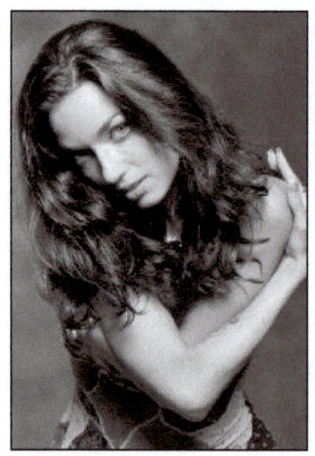

CHAPTER 6

BEST STYLES FOR A ROUND FACE

Synopsis

Prior to even discussing a few dandy styles for round face shapes, you have to understand how to ascertain the shape of your face.

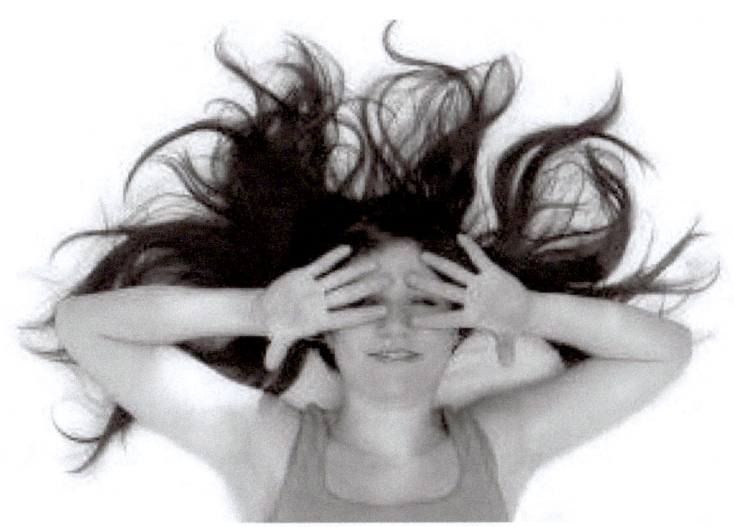

Round

Here is one way to work out your face shape:

To discover the shape of your face, measure it with a tape or ruler. Take (and put down) the accompanying:

- easurements across the top of your cheekbones, then measurements across your jaw line, between the broadest points.

- Measurements across your forehead at the broadest point. Commonly the widest point will be someplace approximately halfway between your eyebrows and your hairline.

- Measurements from the broadest point of your forehead to the bottom of your chin.

There are lots of additional ways women have utilized to figure out this shape -- from sketching the face on a mirror with lipstick to draping it with a towel and asking other people to help figure out the structure.

You are able to try any of these hints or utilize the steps outlined above. Whatever your technique, do remember that this is more about art than scientific discipline!

However whether your face is considered round in the beauty and style region -- or perhaps is more egg-shaped or oblong -- you still have the same destination: to discover the most flattering hairdo possible.

If you've a round face, your face will be approximately as wide as it is long. This might vary a bit where your face isn't quite as wide as it is long, however commonly pretty close.

If you have a round face, you'll have fullness at and beneath your cheekbones. Individuals with round faces likewise tend to have wide hairlines, less-pronounced chins, and their necks frequently appear short.

There truly is no one "perfect" hairdo for a round-shaped face, as a lot of things factor into the total equation. For instance, the length of your hair, its texture and weight, your age and life-style demands all play a part in what is finally the best.

There are great general guideposts that you are able to follow, however the most beneficial solution is to discover a style that works best for you and all your beauty requirements.

If your face is round, the most beneficial hairstyles commonly include:

- Layered bangs instead of flat or heavy bangs.
- Shorter styles which establish height.

- Styles that increase length.

- Styles that keep the sides of your hair shorter or close to the face.

- Curls across the crown -- however never around the cheeks -- to produce height. Keep the sides of your hair shorter with a curly hairdo.

- Longer to really long styles, with bangs and a graduated shag or layers so that the face and the neck are afforded a slimming shape.

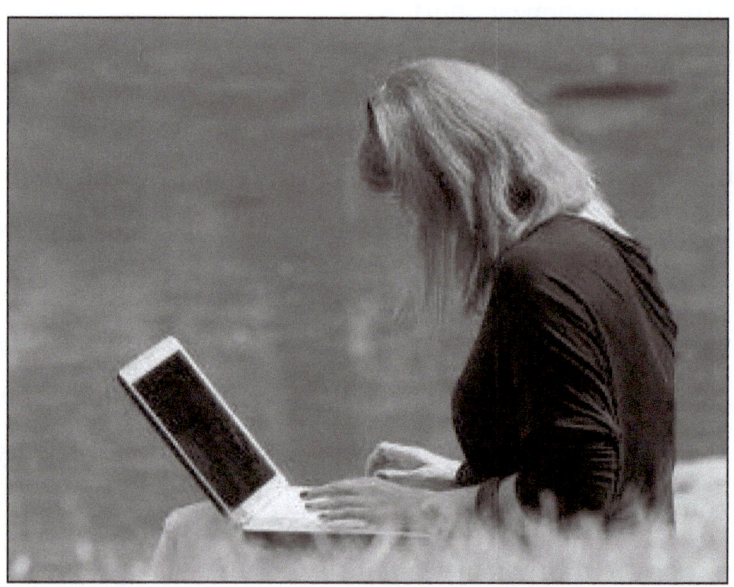

CHAPTER 7

BEST STYLES FOR A HEART SHAPED FACE

Synopsis

Heart-shaped faces are broader at the brow and more narrow at the chin, which commonly adds up to slayer cheekbones. Here, a couple of guideposts for the genetically blessed.

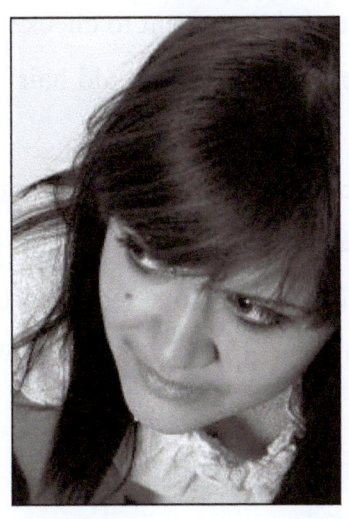

Hearts

Soft, side-swept bangs accent your eyes and draw the focusing away from a pointy chin. Heart-shaped people regularly bring in a photograph of Reese Witherspoon. There's an eroticism and flirtiness about those bangs that each woman in America wishes for. Ask your stylist to trim bangs vertically, instead of straight across, and to stop between the lids and the brows. "If you take them too short, you'll look a little girl.

A long bob that's all one length helps cushion a strong jawline on heart-shaped faces. If you have an exceptional body, you see it - you see the shoulders. And you are able to still tie it up into a ponytail if you go to the gym.

A deep side part brings accent to cheekbones and opens the face up. Finish it up with a flexible-hold hair spray to make your locks look lustrous.

If you desire blunt bangs, make sure to discuss their width with your hairdresser. Cutting bangs at the brows and blending them with faint layers in the front seems to be a hit. You don't need to widen heart-shaped faces any more. When you keep the bangs somewhat narrower, you'll notice the cheekbones, however they won't be so overpowering.

Shoulder-length styles may be dowdy. Loose waves keep the cut young - and draw attention to a strong jaw without looking abrasive. It's reminiscent of Monroe. Using rollers from mid-length to ends to accomplish bounciness is recommended.

Much like a thick side part layers highlight facial characteristics that might be dragged down by longer strands. It's suggested to coax the layers in towards the face with a round brush or flatiron, instead of flipping them out, to keep them appearing modern. This hairdo is best for fine to medium hair, but those with denser hair may ask their stylist to reduce additional bulk utilizing blending shears.

A sleek crop looks sophisticated and fashionable; however it's not for the timid. If you're a heart-shaped face and aren't frightened to show it off, then this is for you. But be aware that it might bring unneeded attention to especially pointy chins.

A bouncy Bob is great for women with flimsier strands. If you raise the hair to this length, it brings fullness. However on other hair sorts, the shape can mushroom cloud. Women with dense or coarse hair ought to avoid it, unless they're going to get a keratin treatment. To get waves, wrap little sections of hair around a one inch curling iron and finish up with a texture cream.

CHAPTER 8

LEARN TO LOVE YOUR STYLE

Synopsis

Would you like to have a hairdo which resembles those of the individuals you see in magazines? If you know what to do, it's conceivable! Here are tricks utilized by many to get their lush, flowing locks. Read on to learn the secrets.

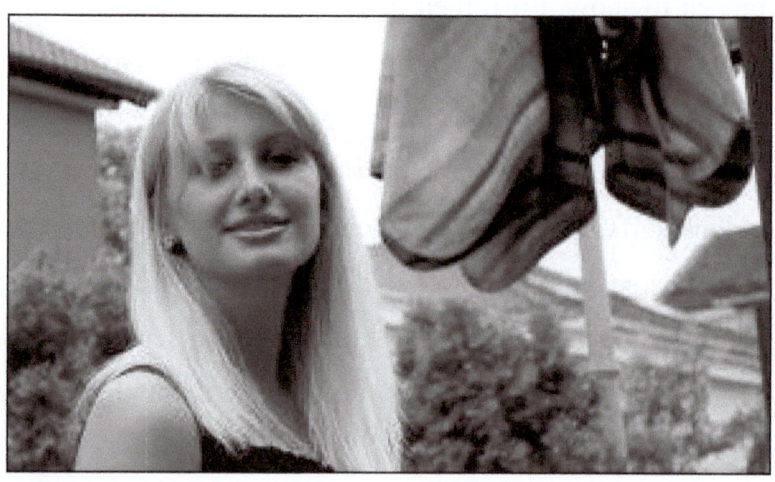

Great Tips

Do you run out of time to fix your hair? You may utilize clips to make your hair look posh. You may put your hair up in an assortment of ways in under 2 minutes.

Dry hair ought to be deep conditioned. If you're suffering with brittle and dry hair, rich conditioning treatment may be done at home by yourself. 1st, simply dampen clean hair. And then apply a rich conditioner, kneading it into your hair. Cover your hair with a cap and let it remain there for up to one-half an hour. Then rinse the conditioner from your hair entirely, let your hair dry naturally and your hair ought to be softer, shinier and more manageable.

There may be a lot of different causes of dandruff. What you might not know is that oily hair may be the culprit. While it might seem counter-intuitive, there's truth behind the statement. Utilize dandruff shampoo or a mild shampoo like baby shampoo to battle dandruff.

Utilize gel in your hair after you twist it. The twist will have a much better appearance and loose hairs will be less likely to break loose. Put a dab of gel onto your finger, and apply it to any scattered hairs. Once these are all attended to, run the tips of your fingers down the twist to get it entirely smooth.

After washing your hair, use a wide-toothed comb and comb out your hair while it's wet. The hair is curliest when wet. Curly hair tends not to tangle as much as straight hair. Abstain from combing your hair too frequently, though, because it may strip your hair of innate oils.

If you're pleased with the appearance of your hair after a dip in the sea, try utilizing hair products that will recreate the effects of seawater. Seek the words "salt spray" on sprays. Attempt putting together a teaspoonful of salt and one cup of water for your own mixture. You ought to then put in around 10 drops of essential lavender oil.

Rub a little bit of olive oil into your hair to keep it glossy. Olive oil moisturizes and shines your hair, which gives it a bright appearance. Place a couple of drops of olive oil in your palm, and rub together before putting it on your hair to keep from producing an oily look.

Dry your hair naturally with a towel, instead of utilizing a blow dryer. The heat a blow dryer produces may damage your hair. If using a towel to dry off your hair, don't be too rigorous, as this may damage and break your hair.

CHAPTER 9

HAIR LOSS TIPS

1. Be healthy for your hair.

When you become healthier, it follows that your hair would have improvements on its health as well. In other words, your hair would also grow faster than usual. Thus, it is best to follow healthy practices, if you want to grow your hair fast, as well as if you want it to look really beautiful.

2. Treat your hair well to make it grow faster.

If you want your hair to grow faster, you have to make sure that it is healthy as well. With that, you have to treat it well, so that it would become as healthy as possible. Treating it well means not using harmful products on it, and caring for it as much as you can each day.

3. Use products that are moisturizing.

Hair that is dry becomes brittle easily, which can also hinder hair growth. Thus, you have to make sure that your hair is full of moisture at all times. With that, you should make sure that you are using moisturizing hair products, such as your shampoos, conditioners, and such.

4. Trim your hair regularly.

You may think that this is counterproductive to hair growth, but, it can really help in speeding up its growth. Trimming means that you cut only about a quarter to a half of an inch of your hair every six weeks or so. By doing this, you can prevent your hair from becoming dry and dull, as well as prevent split ends, which all hinder its growth.

5. Control your stress levels.

Higher stress levels can prevent your hair from growing fast. Thus, it is best to find out ways of relieving yourself from stress. You can do it by getting enough exercise, sleeping well, as well as eating a well balanced diet. Aside from that, going through relaxing activities can also help you out with it.

6. Brushing your hair properly.

Brushing your hair as often as possible can have positive effects on it, especially on its growth. However, there is no need to overdo it, such as the common practice of brushing it for a hundred strokes per night. This is because, this practice can sometimes irritate your scalp, which can result to certain issues, which can prevent proper hair growth.

7. Protect the ends of your hair.

You have to keep in mind that the tips of your hair are the oldest part of it. In other words, the tips are the ones that can get dried out first, which can result to split ends. Thus, you should see to it that the tips are often protected from elements that can put your hair's health at risk. Do not expose it often to the sun, and prevent it from rubbing against the car seat, clothing, and other things that can cause friction.

8. Selecting the right tools for your hair.

Once your hair becomes long enough to style, you may want to make use of certain tools and accessories for it. It is true that these things can make your hair look even more beautiful.

However, you should choose those that are gentle to your hair, so that your hair would retain its health and natural texture.

9. Choosing the right hair styles.

There are hairstyles that necessitate the use of curling iron or a flat iron. These hair styles should be avoided as much as possible, since applying heat on your hair often is not a good idea, when it comes to its health. Choose styles that use simpler methods like twists and wraps, so that you won't put your hair's health at risk.

10. Conditioning your hair.

To ensure that your hair is properly conditioned, whether you are styling it often or not, you should apply a leave on conditioner on it regularly. This type of conditioner will not just make your hair healthier, but it can also protect it from harsh elements. Choose a leave on conditioner that is made by a reputable company to ensure its quality.

11. Don't let heat risk the health of your hair.

It is best to stay away from it as much as you can, for the welfare of your hair. This is because, heat can make your hair dry and brittle, which can prevent it from growing fast. With that, it is best to prevent it from being exposed to the heat of the sun. Aside from that, you should also minimize the use of hair styling tools that give off heat.

12. Protect your hair even at nighttime.

Keep in mind that it is also necessary to protect your hair, even at nighttime. This is because, it is possible that you are rubbing your hair against a pillowcase that can risk its health whenever you are sleeping. To prevent that from happening, you can use a hair cover for it, or make sure that your pillowcase is made out of silk or satin.

13. Use shampoo but not too often.

Using shampoo to your hair is indeed one of the best practices to maintain its health. However, using it too often can actually make it dry, which can result to split ends. Thus, it is best not to shampoo your hair on a daily basis, and do it every other day, so that you can maintain its moisture.

14. Use natural hair care products.

There are lots of hair care products these days, which are loaded with synthetic substances that can harm your locks. With that, it is best to stay away from them, and focus more on using products that are made out of natural substances. Natural hair care products do not contain harmful ingredients, and they are also loaded with vitamins and minerals.

15. Essential fatty acids and zinc.

If you are wondering about what substances can help when it comes to hair growth, then you should take note of zinc and the essential fatty acids. This is because, these substances can prevent dry scalp and dandruff. Thus, by eating foods that contain lots of zinc and fatty acids, you are making your hair healthier, which can encourage its growth.

16. Eating flaxseed.

Flaxseed contain lots of substances that can promote the growth of your hair. Aside from that, it can also make it as shiny as possible. With that, you can add organically milled flax into your daily breakfast meals, such as oatmeal, in order to gain from the benefits that it can offer to you.

17. Swimming pools.

If you love to swim, then you should make use of a hair cap, so that your hair's health won't be at risk. This is because, swimming pools are usually loaded with a lot of chlorine, which can make it unhealthy and dry. There are lots of hair caps that are available today, which can provide adequate protection to your hair. However, it is still best to apply conditioner after every swim, to replenish its lost moisture.

18. Massaging your scalp.

It is true that massaging your scalp on a regular basis can help you achieve faster hair growth. This is because, it can actually stimulate your hair follicles. You can massage your hair while applying conditioner, or just before brushing or styling it, so that you can make it look more beautiful.

19. Eating more fish.

Eating fish is not just healthy, but it can also stimulate hair growth. This is because, fish contains lots of proteins and essential fatty acids, which can improve the health of your hair. With that, it is time that you include fish into your daily meals, so that you can make your hair healthier and grow faster.

20. Shaving your hair.

Some men think that shaving can actually speed up the growth of their hair. However, it actually does not have any effect on hair growth, since hair is just made up of keratin and protein. Thus, shaving it would not make it grow faster. What you can do instead is care for your hair properly, to make it healthier and enhance its growth.

21. Wearing tight hats.

It is not true that tight hats can make you lose lots of hair. However, since a tight hat can increase the temperature around your hair and scalp, wearing it can actually cause damage and breakage to your hair. Thus, if you want to have healthier hair, then make sure that your hat is not too tight. Wear a comfortable one, so that you won't put your hair's health at risk.

22. Dandruff and hair growth.

Dandruff can hinder proper hair growth, since it is caused by a certain type of fungus, which can feed on the oil of your scalp, when it grows out of control. Thus, you should see to it that you follow good hair care methods, which can prevent dandruff. If you have it, then make use of a product that can get rid of it as soon as you can.

23. Withdraw scalp residue.

Withdrawing scalp residue can go a long way, as far as achieving proper hair growth is concerned. This is because, scalp residue can actually clog the hair follicle, which can interfere with the normal growth rate of your hair. To get rid of scalp residue, you can use warm water to wash your scalp, or use apple cider vinegar for it.

24. Warmer climates can result to faster hair growth.

Warmer and humid climates can cause your hair to grow faster. This is because, warm weather can actually help your body produce more oil in your scalp; and, when hair follicles have more natural oils, it can result to faster growth rate. It is best to take note of this, so that you won't try too hard to make your hair grow fast, if you are living in a place that is cold.

25. Increasing blood flow and circulation.

Keep in mind that there are no muscles in between your skull and your scalp. Therefore, blood flow is not as good as the other parts of your body. Increasing the blood flow and circulation in your scalp can stimulate hair growth; and, one of the things you can do for that is to flip your head on each side for 2 to 4 minutes each day.

26. Using rosemary water.

Using rosemary water in washing your hair can stimulate its growth. This is because, it has substances that can stimulate your hair follicles. Aside from that, it also has silicon that can prevent hair loss. Aside from washing your hair with rosemary water though, you can also use it for massaging your scalp.

27. Prevent hair damage to enhance its growth.

If you want to make your hair grow faster, then you should prevent your hair from getting damaged. With that, you should take note of some factors that can cause hair damage. Some of which would be overexposure to the sun, rainwater, dust, certain types of medicines, and such.

28. Drinking rosemary tea.

To promote hair growth, you need to have good blood circulation in your body. Drinking rosemary tea can actually result to proper blood flow. Thus, you can achieve proper hair growth when you drink it. With better blood circulation, your hair would be able to absorb the nutrients it needs to grow.

29. Coloring your hair.

Changing the color of your hair can actually hinder its growth. This is because, hair colors contain substances that can dry out your hair as well as your scalp. Therefore, you should not color your hair often. Aside from damaging your hair, hair colors can also contain toxins, which can also put your health at risk.

30. Using hair gel.

It is true that using hair gel allows you to style your hair according to how you want it to look like. Aside from that, it can also make it shine. However, hair gel is actually sticky, which can result to the accumulation of dust and dirt in your scalp. With that, it can result to dried out hair and scalp in no time, which can prevent your hair from achieving optimum health.

31. Eating eggs.

Eating eggs is one of the best practices, which can enhance the growth of your hair. This is because, eggs are filled with quality protein. Aside from that, they also contain essential B vitamins, iron, zinc, as well as fatty acids, which would all contribute to a healthier hair.

32. Aloe Vera.

The use of Aloe Vera is one of the most popular methods of enhancing the health and growth of hair. You can use it in two ways. First, you can buy hair care products that contain Aloe Vera. On the other hand, you can also obtain an Aloe Vera plant, and apply its juice directly on your scalp.

33. Using Lavender Oil.

Using Lavender Oil on your scalp is one of the best things that you can do in order to boost the health of your hair, and make it grow faster. Massaging your hair with lavender oil would stimulate hair follicles. For maximum results, let the oil stay on your scalp for 30 minutes, before washing it off.

34. Boiling celery leaves and lemon juice.

Applying boiled celery leaves and lemon juice on your scalp can make your hair grow fast. This is because, they contain essential nutrients that can offer that result. Use this mixture after you are done shampooing your hair for a result that you can see in just a matter of weeks.

35. Consume more protein.

Protein is the building blocks of the body, which is why it is essential for proper hair growth and development. With that, it is a good idea to consume foods that are high in protein, so that you can have longer hair in no time. Choose protein sources that are also loaded with other essential nutrients to gain more benefits from it.

Wrapping Up

Having hair like a famous person doesn't call for lots of cash, but lots of work is demanded. Now that you have read the tips in this audiobook, you're aware of gorgeous hair secrets. Take the time to try out these hints and see which ones work for you. Shortly, you'll be the envy of everybody you meet

Printed by Libri Plureos GmbH in Hamburg, Germany